Med School 101
for Patients

Med School 101
for Patients

A Patient's Guide to
Creating an Exceptional Doctor Visit

Kilbourn Gordon III, MD

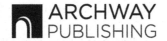
ARCHWAY
PUBLISHING

Archway Publishing books may be ordered through booksellers or by contacting:

Archway Publishing
1663 Liberty Drive
Bloomington, IN 47403
www.archwaypublishing.com
1 (888) 242-5904

Because of the dynamic nature of the Internet, any web addresses or links contained in this book may have changed since publication and may no longer be valid. The views expressed in this work are solely those of the author and do not necessarily reflect the views of the publisher, and the publisher hereby disclaims any responsibility for them.

Any people depicted in stock imagery provided by Thinkstock are models, and such images are being used for illustrative purposes only. Certain stock imagery © Thinkstock.

ISBN: 978-1-4808-4631-9 (sc)
ISBN: 978-1-4808-4632-6 (hc)
ISBN: 978-1-4808-4630-2 (e)

Library of Congress Control Number: 2017942666

Print information available on the last page.

Archway Publishing rev. date: 6/29/2017

I wish a happy and healthy life for all who read this book. What could be more important than excellent health and enjoying life as you move through its different emotional and physical phases? For many of us, our family is our most important ally, supporter, cheering section, and key to good health. Here I celebrate Caroline Britton Gordon, Lindsay Summerill Gordon, Holly Britton Gordon, and Kilbourn Gordon IV: a very special life lived together as a family.

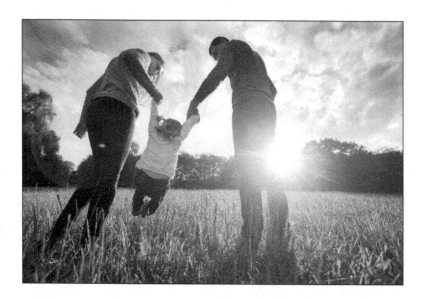

Contents

Foreword

Med School 101 For Patients is a highly readable and informative book that will empower patients to be partners in their care.

Auguste H. Fortin VI, MD, MPH
Professor of Medicine
Director, Medical Interview Curriculum
Yale School of Medicine

Foreword

Highly effective communication around a patient visit to their physician is becoming increasingly important in the current time-sensitive environment of modern medicine. Dr. Gordon, in this highly practical and eminently readable book, provides a most useful guide for navigating before, during, and after that visit. In a step-by-step brass-tacks approach, Dr. Gordon outlines 1) how patients should optimally present the history of their illness, and 2) how patients should ask questions in order to obtain the most useful information in a timely manner. *Med School 101* elevates the quality of the medical office visit to a higher level by emphasizing the importance of an effective partnership between patient and physician in today's medicine, all with an eye toward improving patient care.

Frederick H. Lovejoy Jr., MD
William Berenberg Distinguished Professor of Pediatrics
Harvard Medical School
Associate Physician-in-Chief
Boston Children's Hospital

Acknowledgments

Many people have reviewed the manuscript and provided helpful suggestions, additions, and feedback. I am very thankful for the contributions made by Auguste H. Fortin VI, MD, MPH, Frederick H. Lovejoy Jr., MD, Kym Salness, MD, Michael Glavin, David Tait, Greg Bauer, and my immediate family members.

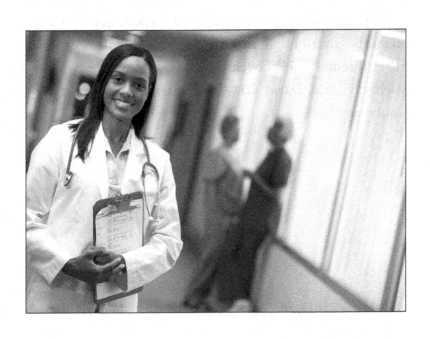

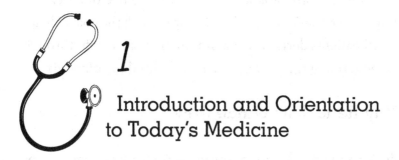

1

Introduction and Orientation to Today's Medicine

Introduction

This book is the product of several years of medical practice experiences. Each day while interacting with patients, one notices very different patient styles. Some patients prefer to be totally receptive to the doctor's thoughts, with few or no questions asked. Other patients ask a multitude of questions.

Each day I am struck by a particularly crisp, succinct question from a patient. Some questions are so well thought out and so well phrased that I compliment the patient with an unofficial "Honorary MD Award." The idea is to reward their logic and quest for knowledge as an essential step in the best possible office visit. They have elevated the visit to a high level of information exchange.

As health care providers, our goal is to ensure the health of all patients and help them to understand their illness along the way. As we work with patients, we notice that some patients are highly motivated to uncover the correct diagnosis and therapy.

Why can't all patients have the experience of an exceptional office visit? This book was written with the goal of helping all patients derive the maximum medical benefit through understanding the process and logic behind the office visit.

Why Read This Guide Now?

Modern medicine encompasses a massive amount of data derived by multiple caregivers.

Physical findings, test results, imaging studies, medication data—the amount of information entered into the electronic medical record is continuously growing. The types and numbers of health care workers are also growing: nurses, specialists, pharmacists, physical therapists. The net result is that the amount of medical information for a specific patient has grown exponentially. The volume of information is so large that it can be difficult to coordinate and prioritize the importance of a specific data point for a specific patient. At the same time, the ability to identify which parts of the data are significant is an essential skill for unlocking the true nature of a patient's illness.

Medicine has to be delivered in a highly efficient manner these days.

Due to reimbursement cutbacks, many physicians are having difficulty paying their overhead and keeping their practices open. Therefore, they must see more patients in a shorter amount of time.

Your first reaction to the present medical environment might be that you, the patient, could be shortchanged by this setting. This book is intended to help you respond to this changing landscape by understanding how you can help yourself receive better outcomes within these shorter visits.

Such a condensed medical office visit can be just as productive as a longer visit. However, you the patient must ensure that your essential questions are answered and unknown aspects are identified.

Your personal time with your health care professional comes down to a matter of a few minutes: perhaps just ten or fifteen minutes. Everything that happens during this session is important: how you have prepared (or not prepared) for the session, what records you have kept regarding your illness, what questions you will ask, and what education regarding your condition you expect to receive from your caregiver.

Medicine is increasingly characterized by the supreme importance of accurate diagnosis and treatment.

The advent of modern testing and imaging studies in addition to rigorous training for doctors—these are rooted in the need to uncover the truth for each patient. In addition, medicine practiced in the United States is intensely scrutinized by lawyers whose professional goal is to generate malpractice lawsuits. Accurate diagnosis and treatment is crucial to the welfare of both patient and doctor.

Medicine is delivered by multiple types of health care professionals who have learned their skills through very different training.

Doctors are only part of the team, which also includes physicians' assistants (PA) and advanced practical registered nurses (APRNs, also known as nurse practitioners). Before you enter the room for your evaluation, you should be aware of who will be evaluating you and the type of training they have undertaken. PAs have attended PA school, which is approximately a two-year program following a college degree. APRNs have graduated from nursing school and have attended an additional two years of training.

Medicine is now fully computerized, with all medical records (so called EMR: electronic medical records) handled by computer.

Although this clearly permits simplified ability to look up prior medical information, it also requires that the physician input data during the process of the visit (some practitioners do all their EMR charting following the patient visit). When the EMR is completed in the presence of the patient, it takes time and attention from the needs of the patient.

Completion of an EMR chart for each patient visit is an extra step in the process, which physicians did not have to address just a few years ago. The process takes extra cognitive energy, energy that could be used to help you, the patient. In a perfect world, the patient would be the recipient of all diagnostic and therapeutic energies. However, the extra EMR step in the visit process leaves less energy for the patient. You must be aware of this limitation in order for you to improve your visit.

Caregiver Overview

You may have noticed that your care is provided by not only doctors but also by nurse practitioners and physicians assistants. Given the large need for primary care in the United States, both nurse practitioners and physician assistants are filling the void. Because all three types of professionals give care, they are referred to, collectively, as providers. In this booklet, we may use the word physician as our provider, but the same concepts can be used for care given by nurse practitioners and physician assistants.

All three types of providers are subject to the daily stresses of medical practice. We must understand their inherent biases and their decision-making processes.

Present-Day Health Care Overview

Medical practice has undergone dramatic changes in the past twenty-five years. Once considered as people of great respect and dignity, doctors have become commoditized service providers. Commoditized serviced providers are viewed as interchangeable managers of patient care. As an example of this, we note that patients readily switch from doctor to doctor, depending on their insurance coverage. Patients would like to be loyal to their doctor, but financial considerations often hinder these longstanding relationships. Another example is that your PCP may not be available to see you on a specific day, and you may be assigned to a physician you do not know.

Doctors remain an essential ingredient in providing an essential service. The difference in modern medicine is that doctors are seen as replaceable and interchangeable. The commoditization of doctoring has relegated doctors to be viewed as everyday participants of an essential people service: the practice of medicine.

Within the backdrop of medical service commoditization, two components remain unchanged: the ongoing patient needs of both an accurate diagnosis and an effective therapy. Patients will continue to need and deserve the best possible care, regardless of how their caregivers are viewed by the medical system and their patients.

How do we arrive at accurate diagnoses and effective therapies given the backdrop of radical medical practice changes? The answer is that you the patient must take on new roles and responsibilities. You must make an effort to know your doctor on a very personal level: their medical training, their inherent biases, their personal situation, and their approach to practicing medicine. In short, we need to understand our doctors as people who have biases, limitations, and emotions. We need to push back the commoditization of medicine by treating our physicians as the intricate people they are. We need to accept them as human beings, people who are trying to provide the best care possible in an extremely challenging environment.

By making the effort to understand his or her personal

side, you are showing your doctor that you care for them as well. The setting of mutual respect and personal understanding of each person's situation creates a powerful dynamic. It is the key tenet of this guide that mutual respect and understanding between doctor and patient creates an entirely new level of honesty and clarity of medical decision making. Accurate diagnoses and most effective therapies will naturally flow from this relationship.

You might think to yourself, *This is obvious: mutual respect and understanding creates better care.* If this appears obvious to you, just think back to the last time you asked your doctor to discuss their challenges within modern-day medicine, their training, their inherent biases, and their personal life. The medical visit is traditionally characterized by almost all emphasis on the patient and his or her condition. We propose that now is the time for you, the patient, to change this outdated approach and create new understanding that flows naturally with your doctor.

The Importance of Primary Care Physician (PCP)

Your primary care physician knows you better than any other health care provider. They are in a unique position to guide your care, provide perspective on your present situation, and help you to decide next steps. Listen to them carefully. Their only goal is to restore you to full health. They are your partner in pursuit of excellent health.

Primary care is the entry point for your care. The basic

laboratory tests and imaging will be done here. An analysis of your situation will be discussed. You must be in the right frame of mind to complement the skills of your PCP: be open to their perspective. You must fully understand their thinking and their concerns. They are your best friend in the pursuit of helping yourself. Given that most common medical problems can be determined from the basic medical history and physical exam, the PCP is the cornerstone of your care.

The primary care physician is uniquely positioned to look at all of your symptoms, even if they are located in different organ systems. Your primary care physician is the one physician that knows all aspects of you. You must actively provide all the tools they need to help you by optimizing the office visit.

Disease Overview: Categories

It is important to have a basic understanding of disease so you can explain your situation to your doctor with some basic background knowledge.

Disease is the state of abnormal functioning at the cellular level. As the problem becomes more manifest and larger numbers of cells are affected, it begins to affect our daily lives. Let us look specifically at each form of disease.

Infectious Disease

Infectious disease is the situation when an outside bacteria, virus, or fungus invades your body, thereby disrupting normal processes. A simple example is Streptococcus Group A bacteria invading our tonsils to create fever in the setting of strep throat.

Metabolic Disease

Metabolic disease is a derangement in the normal chemical processes of the body. An example is one form of diabetes mellitus in which the amount of insulin is reduced, resulting in the inability of the cells to use glucose and the resultant high blood glucose levels.

Genetic Disease

Genetic disease is based on DNA abnormalities such that anatomic and/ or metabolic abnormalities are present. A well-known example is Down syndrome with its cognitive impairments and anatomic defects such as heart abnormalities.

Anatomic Disease

Anatomic disease is a derangement of the normal anatomy, such that normal processes are disrupted. An example is kidney stones whose size and shape block the normal flow of urine within the urinary system. We can also think in terms of organ system failure: liver failure, renal failure. In each of these organs, the specialized cells within the organ demonstrate abnormal function.

Cancer

Cancer is an additional disease category. It is characterized by the emergence of abnormal cells where previously normal cells were present. These cells replicate very quickly and often disrupt normal functioning. Cancer has two major forms: solid tumors (think of a lung tumor expanding as it grows within the lung) and blood-borne cancers such as leukemias (white cells growing at such a fast rate that they interfere with many aspects of normal blood function).

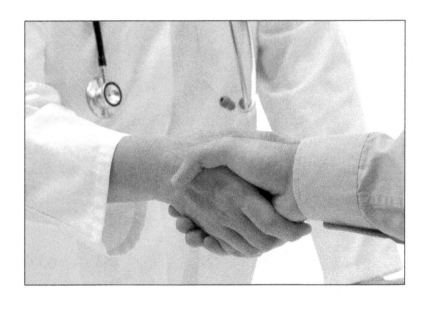

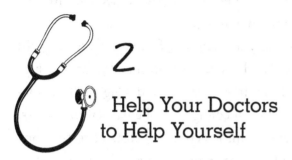

2
Help Your Doctors to Help Yourself

Help your doctors in order to help yourself. The premise of this book is that doctors need your help to make the best decisions for your medical care. Your extra efforts will create an exceptional office visit with the goal of accurate diagnosis and effective therapies.

Doctors are people just like you. All of us experience difficulties with making decisions, and we experience stress on the job. Many of us perform work-related duties that are subject to limitations imposed by other workers. However, doctors have additional decision-making challenges and are constantly subject to stressful situations. Doctors' decisions affect people's health and well-being. Increasingly they are subject to a multitude of bureaucratic requirements imposed by insurance companies, health systems, and hospitals. Sadly, these restrictions leave less time for the most important part of their profession: you, the patient.

Doctors have spent many years learning their trade from both books and patients. During these many years, their singular goal has been to perform excellent medical care, utilizing excellent decision making.

After years of daily academic information exchange in both medical school and residency training, doctors are supposedly free to make their own decisions during medical practice. However, this has all changed in the past twenty years. Doctors must now take into account all sorts of restrictions and liability considerations. Some examples of these externally imposed structures include medical treatment protocols, insurance company rules, pharmacy benefit manager limits on drug selection, and required electronic medical record use. In addition, hospitals, the residence of the sickest patients, enforce additional rules and regulations.

Given this daunting situation, your doctor is challenged in more ways than at any prior time in the history of medicine. Providing the best possible care has never been more difficult.

Traditional Western medical thinking as practiced over the past many years is exemplified by a predictable series of events. You go to the doctor, they evaluate you, they decide the diagnosis, and they decide the appropriate treatment. This one-way evaluation and treatment is not only outdated but is potentially detrimental to your health.

Making decisions within medicine is complicated. Within this book, we will identify many of the factors that can lead to incorrect diagnosis and treatment. By becoming an active participant in the process of the office visit, you are most likely to have an optimal medical outcome.

In the past few years, a new partnership has emerged between caregiver and patient. During the visit, you, the patient, start by providing the caregiver with relevant data as in the traditional office visit. After this traditional information exchange, the dynamics of the partnership change quickly. You, the patient, assume an active role by participating in the medical decision process through highly relevant probing questions and other partnership sharing techniques.

The key to unlocking the best attributes of your doctor is to understand how they think, understand their challenges, and help them with the medical decision-making process. Help your doctor to help yourself.

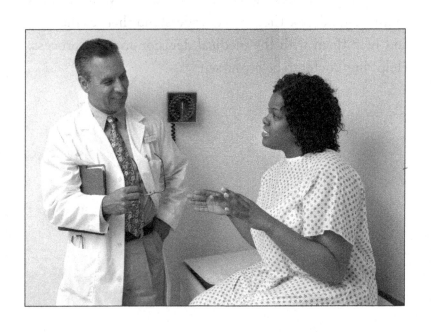

Patient as Partner with Doctor in Providing Health Care

The core tenet of this new philosophy is that the patient and the physician are active participating partners with each other during the office visit. Each side has an equal level of interest, participation, responsibility, and ownership of the process. Each has the direct and immediate goal of attaining your best health care. Active engagement of each side is an inherent component to the success of the other; cooperation is the key to exceptional health care.

The patient must be prepared for the visit. This includes having thought through all the essential elements of their condition, considered questions appropriate to ask, and considered the timing of the questions. The physician must ask the relevant questions as to the onset of the illness and accompanying symptoms, synthesize the data presented, and formulate one or more diagnoses. It is crucial that patient and physician are equally engaged in both inquiry and providing information. The interactions by and between the patient and physician govern the outcome of their meeting with major consequences as to a positive or negative result.

The word "patient," when used as a noun, describes a person who is undergoing medical treatment. The same word "patient," when used as an adjective, describes a person who is uncomplaining, calm, quiet, and passive. Therefore, a patient patient is a person undergoing medical treatment who remains passive throughout the doctor visit and accepts the outcomes as presented. Since the goal of this book is to transform you, the patient, into an active participant within the entire process, we propose a new name for you: "patient partner."

Think of yourself as a patient partner, with an emphasis on the word "partner." As you read this guide, start to assimilate the approach we present; understand your new role as one half of a highly effective two-member team. See yourself as a mobilized, empowered, and contributing individual with a health condition that requires the very best medical evaluation and treatment.

Attitude is everything: a partnership implies mutual respect, cordial discussion, debate, and a large helping of kindness and gratitude. The ability to establish the partnership, work through the problem, specify the plan together during a short ten-minute visit, is the goal you share.

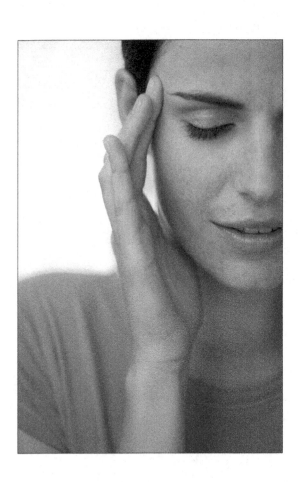

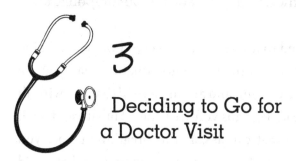

3

Deciding to Go for a Doctor Visit

Perhaps you have been sick for a day, for three days, or for a month. When should you seek an evaluation?

Fever

Fever is usually the sign of a significant infection. Sometimes these are viral infections that are treated symptomatically, but other times they are bacterial infections for which antibiotics should be considered. Because it is difficult to determine viral versus bacterial etiology, your physician should be consulted.

Pain

You are uncomfortable on account of pain: sudden onset of new pain could signal that something significant inside your body has become problematic. For example, chest pain may signal heart attack, and thus immediate care should be sought. Any and all abdominal pain is significant and should be evaluated by your health care professional.

Unstable situation with potential to decompensate.

You are concerned that your situation could worsen, causing you to be in a much more precarious situation than you are now. Perhaps you feel faint and are concerned that you will fall and hurt your head. Perhaps you are short of breath and want to be in a facility that can assist your breathing before you are unable to breathe. Perhaps you have chest pain that could decompensate into an arrhythmia, which could be treated successfully in a health care facility.

You do not feel well.

Your energy is decreased, and you are not sure why this is happening to you. Fatigue is a common problem and requires a full physical exam along with laboratory testing.

Ongoing monitoring.

You are aware that ongoing problems such as high blood pressure and diabetes must be monitored in order to prevent complications. You desire monitoring and modification of treatment when appropriate.

Loss of function.

You are having a problem with normal everyday activities but cannot explain why this is happening to you. For example, you used to remember where the extra toothbrushes were kept, but now you cannot find them. Any loss of function, whether it be motor function such as walking or sensory functions such as seeing, will be distressing to you and require explanation and treatment.

Okay, now you have decided to go for an evaluation. This book is organized in a sequential manner that parallels the experience you have with your doctor. Let us discuss the structure of the guide in order to aid you with the process.

The Structure of *Med School 101* Reflects the Structure of the Medical Visit

This book is divided into three distinct parts: 1) pre-visit preparation; 2) within-visit medical history review, physical exam, discussion; and 3) post-visit next steps. Pre-visit preparation includes the nuts and bolts of which data will be required at the visit. Within-visit processing includes: 1) a detailed discussion of medical history; 2) a detailed physical exam; and 3) discussion of diagnosis and treatment. Post-visit next steps provide patients with the ability to review the findings and create a strategy for answering difficult questions going forward.

During the process of the visit, you should be asking yourself, where am I in the process? How prepared am I for each part of the process?

Med School 101 is written in a small book format on purpose. You can bring the book with you to your visit and refer to it when needed. In addition, you can show your physician certain concepts and questions that are discussed in the book.

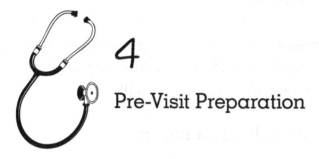

4
Pre-Visit Preparation

You know that during your visit you will be asked lots of questions regarding your condition, your medication, your past medical history, and lots of other background information. In this section, we will examine each one of these areas and develop your personal information packet. It is possible that your doctor's website has a template for this information, so be sure to check it before you start this section.

We are going to discuss each aspect of the information packet from the perspective of the doctor. Our discussion is based on the way that all physicians are taught to perform the history and physical. If you know how the doctor thinks about your situation from their prior training and their usual intake of information, then you are more likely to have the best medical outcome.

We suggest you write down your specific information for each of the following components of the medical history.

1. Chief Complaint

The chief complaint is the reason you are going for your evaluation. It is expressed in just a few words. An example is: "Pain of the left ankle after twisting it on a sidewalk."

2. History of the Present Illness

This area describes all aspects of your present problem. When did it start? What makes it better or worse? What time of day do the symptoms arise? How have the symptoms changed over time? What treatments have been tried and what were their effects? What labs or imaging studies have already been performed? What have other doctors determined as the diagnosis, and what was their thinking about other possible reasons for the problem?

Detail is important here. Very small clues can help discover the true reason for your problem. Think carefully about all aspects of your medical condition and write them down. Describe the condition with great attention to detail. For example, when describing pain, discuss the nature of the pain: intermittent, constant, searing, electrical, dull, throbbing, or any other best descriptor you can imagine. Does the pain start in one place and move to another?

3. Past Medical and Surgical History

All of your prior medical conditions should be listed here. These include hypertension, diabetes, gout, heart disease, and all other conditions. All surgeries should be documented and should include the year the surgery was performed if known to you.

4. Medications

Each medication you are taking should be documented. The dosage amount and number of times per day you take the medicines should be mentioned. Over-the-counter medicines are important as well.

5. Allergies to Medicines

Any problems you have had with prior medicines should be described here. True allergies would include symptoms such as hives and shortness of breath. However, drugs can have side effects that are intolerable, even though they might not be true allergies. For example, a specific antibiotic might give a patient a stomach ache, even though it would be otherwise safe to take the medicine. This section should really be labeled as "Troubles with Medicine," as it includes true allergies as well as any and all problems you have experienced with medicine. In reality, all prior troubles with medicine are discussed under this section.

6. Social History

This section deals with your consumption of alcohol and tobacco. You should specify how many packs of cigarettes you smoke per day and for how many years you have smoked. The number of alcoholic drinks per day should be documented. In addition, marital status is documented.

7. Family History

Think carefully about the major medical problems that have been present in your family. Specify which of your siblings, parents, or grandparents have had any of the following conditions: heart disease, cancer, stroke, diabetes or any other major disease.

You have completed your homework on paper. Now it is time to prepare for the visit itself by practicing the "presentation" of your case.

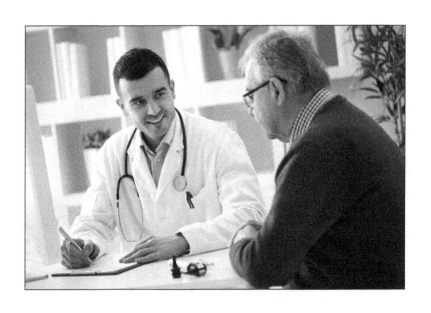

Presentation of Your Case: Practice Prior to Visit

During medical school and residency training, doctors are constantly discussing patients with each other. This enables them to compare thinking, workups, diagnosis, and therapy. They start this process by presenting the patient's case to another doctor or group of doctors in a meeting. The presentation of a patient case is a very formal process with a specific order in which the patient data is discussed. It starts with the following phrase:

"Mrs. Jones is a fifty-eight-year-old female with a three-day history of abdominal pain" (this is the chief complaint we have discussed above). The process then continues along the path we have outlined above: 2) history of the present illness, 3) past medical and surgical history, 4) medications, 5) allergies to medications, 6) social history, 7) family history. This is the first half of the presentation; it is followed by the vital signs and a discussion of the complete head-to-toe physical examination.

Let us then give an example of the first half of the presentation for Mrs. Jones. It might go like this:

"Mrs. Jones is a fifty-eight-year-old female with a three-day history of right lower quadrant abdominal pain made worse by walking and the bumps in the road, accompanied by two days of vomiting and diarrhea. The pain is accompanied by fever, chills, and backache. Mrs. Jones returned from Nicaragua two days before the pain started. Her past medical history is significant for diabetes and hypertension. Her surgical history is significant for an appendectomy age twenty-one. Her medications include atenolol for hypertension and metformin for diabetes. She is allergic to penicillin. Her social history includes smoking for twenty years, one pack per day, and social drinking of alcohol. Her mother has breast cancer and her father has diabetes."

We suggest that you rehearse the presentation of your case prior to the medical visit. Be ready to deliver the presentation with all the elements listed above. Start your presentation with: "I am fifty-eight years old with a three-day history of ..." This approach will surely cause your doctor to pay the utmost attention. You are feeding him data in the same way that his doctor colleagues talk to him. You are presenting your case in a way that is efficient and is compatible with patient data transfer that is a core part of medical training. You have elevated yourself and your case to high attention status.

Before discussing the visit itself, we must review some areas of caution.

A Note of Caution: Pre-Visit Preparation Includes Careful Thought as to What Events During the Visit Could Be Problematic

Given that you will be operating in a more robust role than most patients, it is of paramount importance that you nurture your relationship with your doctor from the very beginning of the encounter. You must make them feel good about themselves and their role. You must keep them in your court as your best advocate. You must ensure that they are fully committed to creating a partnership with you. How do you do this?

Begin the medical visit by saying that you want to be more involved in the process than most patients. You want to help the doctor in all possible ways. You will be asking a few more questions than most patients, but you understand that the doctor has time limitations and you will work within these limitations.

Think of the medical visit as a ten-minute session (six hundred seconds), where all aspects of the medical visit must be covered. Thus, you will need to cover all the basic information (the history and physical exam) in the first five minutes. This will give you five minutes for the all-important discussion and decision-making phase. If the office has allotted fifteen minutes for the visit, then you will have more than ten minutes for the decision-making portion. In order for the history and physical phase to take only five minutes, you will have to expedite the process by your thorough preparation and knowledge of what will take place.

If you challenge the doctor's thinking excessively (excessive numbers of questions or excessive amount of time required), you may be viewed as a problem patient. This is the exact antithesis of our desired result. You can avoid this outcome and ensure effective patient outcome by giving the doctor an out early in the process.

Here is a concrete suggestion: After introducing yourself and your proposed robust effective patient role, just say that you will curb your questions if they seem excessive to the doctor. Mention that you realize that they work under strict time limitations. Pay attention to the doctor's response at all times. If their answer seems short or curt, they are probably feeling uncomfortable, and you should give them the option to move forward.

In short, you must gain the trust of the doctor. Introduce them to your robust new patient role and explain your reasoning: you want to help the doctor and yourself to more efficiently arrive at quality care. Ensure they feel good about the process before continuing further. Think about your office visit as similar to taking an academic test: prepare well, work within the allotted time, and have all essential questions answered.

Your goal for the visit is to derive an accurate diagnosis regarding your condition and to understand the treatment options available to you. In order to reach this goal, we want you to personally be involved in the process of the visit. The more you understand the process and the more you work within this process, the closer you are to successful resolution of your medical problem.

You have done your homework, prepared well for the visit, and thought through potential problems. Let us now discuss the visit itself.

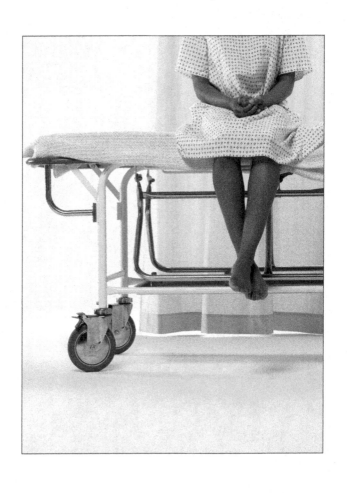

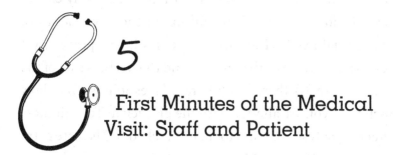

5

First Minutes of the Medical Visit: Staff and Patient

The first component of the process is to introduce yourself and establish a positive rapport with the medical assistant or nurse. The medical assistant or nurse is the staff member who brings you back to the examination room and asks the initial questions. Their job is to obtain a brief outline of the chief complaint. In addition, they will obtain the past medical and surgical histories, your present medicines, your allergies, social history, and family history. After completing the basic questions, they will check your vital signs: temperature, blood pressure, pulse rate, respiratory rate, and pulse oximetry (the noninvasive measurement of oxygen in your blood). The medical assistant or nurse has "warmed you up" prior to the physician entering the room. This permits everyone to be on the same page; your information is provided to the doctor through the electronic medical record before he or she walks in the examination room.

Of special note is that the medical assistant or nurse has the ear of the physician. Thus, if you need something special to be done (such as a quick visit, form filled out, call to pharmacy), the medical assistant or nurse will likely ensure that this does happen. They will tip off the physician as to your special needs. They are your allies in the process, yet they participate on both your side and the doctor's side of the visit. You can ask them candid, frank questions, such as how much time you are allotted with the physician. Ten minutes? Fifteen minutes? Is the doctor behind schedule? Is there extra time allotted if needed? Do they work through lunch hour to catch up to the set schedule?

Now present your case to the medical assistant or nurse. It includes all the information they must record prior to the arrival of the doctor. Your presentation is the exact information they need to complete your chart.

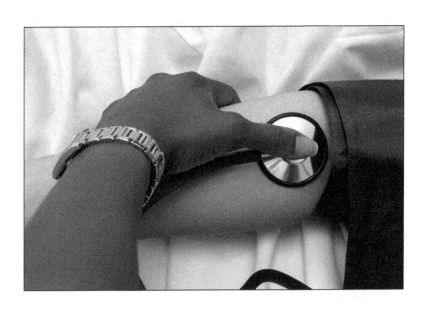

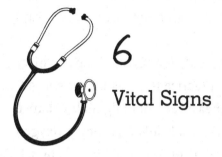

6

Vital Signs

Vital signs include blood pressure, pulse, temperature, and pulse oximetry. Let us discuss each one of these measurements.

Blood pressure can be normal, high, or low. High blood pressure is a risk for heart disease and stroke. Low blood pressure can be an ominous sign: shock and impending death may be imminent.

Pulse is the measure of heart beats per minute. A heart rate over one hundred is called tachycardia. Some tachycardias are not immediately harmful (fever, dehydration), but others can be very harmful (ventricular tachycardia) and life threatening. All tachycardias deserve to be addressed as to their cause in order to assess risk.

A heart rate below sixty beats per minute is called a bradycardia. Very low heart rates below fifty beats per minute can result in fainting and should be addressed. Low heart rates can be due to extensive training, as in marathon runners, or due to intrinsic heart disease. Once again, understanding the underlying cause is of utmost importance.

Temperature is important as a gauge of infectious disease

severity. A fever is any temperature above 100.4. High fever is indeed worrisome, and a search for its cause is always warranted.

Pulse oximetry is a new vital sign. Over the past thirty years, it has become routine practice to measure oxygen saturation by the noninvasive measurement of light absorbance through a patient's finger. Normal pulse oximetry oxygen saturation values are in the range of 97–99 percent. Low saturation values indicate problems with lung function, such as pneumonia or asthma.

You have presented your case to the medical assistant or nurse as a rehearsal for the presentation to the doctor. Once the medical assistant or nurse has recorded your information in the computer, your vital signs will be taken. Utilize the available time before the doctor enters the room to review your case presentation once again.

Think carefully as to the specific elements of the history of the present illness. When did your condition start? Did something happen to cause this? What makes it worse? What makes it better? If it is pain, where does it radiate? Does it come and go? What other problems are you experiencing at the same time: fever, chills, vomiting, diarrhea, sore throat, malaise?

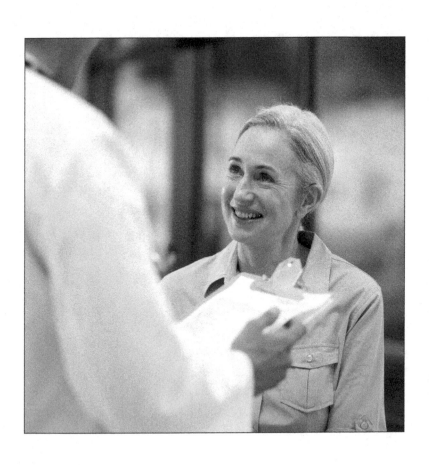

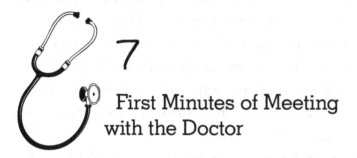

7

First Minutes of Meeting with the Doctor

When the physician enters the room, introduce yourself. After saying your name, you might mention a personal anecdote: "My mother enjoyed being your patient just last week," or, "My neighbor has told me that this is a very personal and thorough medical practice." Just a one- or two-sentence chitchat about something you have noticed will place you on the same discussion plane as your doctor. If you are indeed aware of something positive regarding the practice, your mention of it has the effect of upping the ante as to a quality visit. This is a key element of the visit: you need the doctor to be your partner in the pursuit of your correct diagnosis and treatment. Positive comments are special words to the doctor. You have acknowledged that you respect the doctor and want to work with him or her. Most patients do not start with these comments.

Your approach is different. It is personal, attentive, and positive. These are likely to be the same attributes you hope to be present in your doctor's approach to you and your illness. Any great partnership starts with mutual respect, trust, and an alignment of values. Think of the beginning seconds of the visit as an opportunity to set the stage for a great partnership. Start by exemplifying the values you wish to see in your provider.

The formal beginning of the doctor-patient interaction is your presentation of your medical history directly to the doctor. This is the time when you give the presentation that you have rehearsed at home prior to the visit and presented to the medical assistant or nurse.

Remember the order of items to be discussed: this is the checklist we discussed earlier. Start with the chief complaint, then discuss the history of the present illness, your past medical and surgical history, your medications, your allergies to medications, your social history (tobacco, alcohol, and marital status), and family history. This is your chance to provide relevant detail regarding your history. All of the historical components discussed above can help you. However, the chief complaint and history of the present illness are the two most important data points for your visit.

Many diagnoses can be determined by just the medical history and physical exam. Your detailed yet quick description of the history is your greatest opportunity to contribute to the successful outcome of the visit. Your rehearsal of the presentation of your case at home and just prior to the entrance of the doctor will make this section easy for you and a welcome addition for the doctor.

Additionally, it is highly advised that at the beginning of the visit, you state very clearly your agenda: your needs, your concerns, and the answers you are looking for. A recent patient visit in my practice illustrates the importance of voicing your concerns early on in the visit. Let us describe this patient in detail.

A fifty-four-year-old female with a three-day history of left shoulder pain presented to our office. The pain was worse with movement and could be reproduced with pressure on the muscles of the shoulder. Without knowledge of the patient's concerns, I decided to perform an electrocardiogram to ensure that the shoulder pain was not caused by a subtle heart attack. After discussing the normal EKG with the patient, she said, "I am very relieved that you took an EKG. I read on the Internet that shoulder pain can be a heart attack."

A better scenario would have been if the patient described her symptoms in the usual manner and then proceeded to explain that she was concerned about a heart attack and wanted an EKG to help diagnose the origin of the chest pain. It is best for you, the patient, to voice such concerns and expectations at the beginning of the office visit, immediately after the doctor enters your exam room.

During this medical history review, your doctor is likely to simultaneously ask you questions and record your answers in a nearby computer. Just at the very time you are hoping to converse directly with your doctor, they appear to be utilizing most of their energy to input your data into the computer. This situation can be rather disconcerting to both you and the doctor. A simple comment from you to acknowledge this awkward situation will improve the situation. You might say to your doctor, "Gosh, it must take a lot of energy to input all that data about me and also be able to make medical decisions at the same time." This signals that you are hoping for a more personal and direct, eye-to-eye interaction.

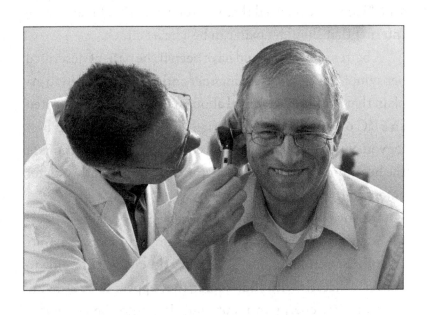

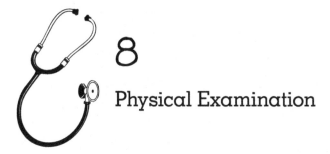

8
Physical Examination

The second phase of the office visit is the physical exam. This is the part of the visit where the physician examines you using all of his or her tools: pushing and prodding, tapping on specific areas, feeling for heat or coolness of areas, examining for pulses, testing for normal sensation, and listening for the sounds of the heart, lung, and bowels. Your body will often be examined in an orderly manner: head first, toes last for a complete bodily exam.

Your contribution during this stage is minimal. You simply sit or lie down and permit the examination. However, your responses to being examined are important. Where exactly was the most pain felt when the doctor pushed on you? What kind of pain was it: dull, sharp, electric? Did pushing on the painful area make it worse or have no effect?

The physical exam will most likely be tailored to the area of the body that relates to the symptoms. For example, a patient presenting with cough and cold will likely have head, ear, eyes, nose, throat, and lungs examined, and the rest of the body will likely remain unexamined.

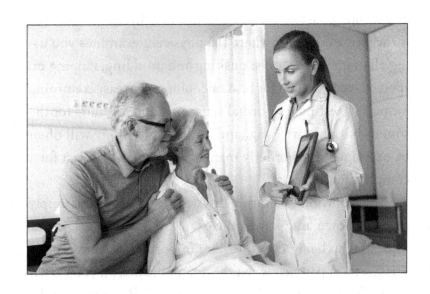

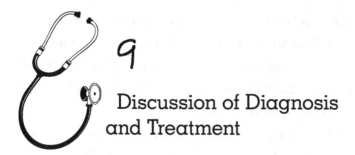

9

Discussion of Diagnosis and Treatment

The third stage of the visit is the discussion phase where the diagnosis and treatment are discussed. We are going to discuss diagnosis and treatment in extensive detail because these are the pivotal decision components of your visit. They are also the keys to unlocking your return to health. Let us first discuss diagnosis.

Diagnosis and Differential Diagnosis

Determining an accurate diagnosis is no small task. It involves critical thinking with analysis of all aspects of the patient: the chief complaint, the history of the present illness, the past medical and surgical history, allergies, medications, social history, family history, physical exam, and recent testing. It is a very complex process, requiring the synthesis of large amounts of patient-specific data viewed within the backdrop of all possible medical conditions.

The task of building a list of all possible relevant medical conditions is called the differential diagnosis. If a physician is unaware of a specific medical condition (because it was not included in their training, their reading, or their prior experience), they will not include that specific diagnosis in their differential diagnosis. The stakes are high for a missed diagnosis when the differential diagnosis is incomplete and dangerous conditions are present.

You and I as patients think in terms of a single diagnosis, a single condition that is causing us to be sick. Doctors are trained, however, to think in terms of differential diagnosis: a list of *all* potential causes of the condition. This term, differential diagnosis, illuminates the possible diagnoses under one umbrella. For a given symptom, such as a rash, there are many different diagnoses; that is, there are many different possible underlying causes of the rash with many different mechanisms. Therefore, the hard truth is that there may be a number of potential causes for a specific medical problem. Each underlying cause is indeed a different diagnosis.

The good news is that most common maladies are so common that they are easy to diagnose correctly. It is important for your own health, however, to understand how the physician thinks in order to help ensure accuracy of diagnosis and treatment. A deeper understanding of medical decision making is of paramount importance, even given an apparently easy, quick diagnosis.

A single symptom could be caused by one of many underlying disease processes. For example, a rash on the leg could be the result of the following:

1. An allergic reaction to something that touched the area

2. An infectious disease that is present within the whole body, such as Lyme disease
3. An infection of the skin by a bacteria called cellulitis
4. A coagulation disorder resulting in bleeding under the skin

In this example, the initial diagnosis is rash, but the more specific diagnosis gives us an indication of the underlying mechanism and therefore treatment. In the present example, the more specific diagnosis could be any one of the following: 1) allergic reaction, 2) Lyme disease, 3) cellulitis, and 4) hematoma.

Now that you understand how a doctor thinks about your symptoms, let's discuss how you can obtain a window into their more detailed thought process. It is very important to consider how you ask your question. If you ask, "What is the differential diagnosis?" you sound like you are the doctor and are trying to usurp his or her thinking. You do not want to undermine the confidence and partnership you have built over time with each other. You would like to know the entire list of diagnoses, but this detailed list may not be right on the tip of his or her tongue. To avoid alienating your doctor, simply say, "What are the most likely things that could be causing my illness?"

After a brief discussion of each specific diagnosis, it will be important to prioritize the list with regards to the potential for short-term harm to the patient. Thus, you might consider asking an additional question that begins to uncover the risks involved to you personally within each diagnosis. For example, you might say, "Are any of these causes particularly danger-ous? Is there a critical time factor for any of these conditions?"

Exact Diagnosis: Probably Problematic

When you go to your physician for an evaluation, you enter the experience thinking that you will be coming home with an exact diagnosis. With simple conditions such as coughs and colds, this is indeed often the situation. However, the exact diagnosis is not always obvious on the first visit. The elusive exact diagnosis may require testing to assist the deci-sion, may require repeated examinations over time to monitor how things develop, or may require a visit to the specialist to identify rare conditions.

You may leave the doctor's office feeling unnerved or even a little bit more scared than when you entered. Our message is that those feelings are appropriate and provide motivation for continuing the search for the definitive diagnosis.

Each day, doctors are faced with situations that do not per-mit specification of an exact diagnosis. This is not an uncom-mon situation. It is of utmost importance to your health that you, the patient, are willing to accept this and be comfortable with developing a strategy to pinpoint an accurate diagnosis in conjunction with your doctor.

Work as a partner with your doctor to improve the infor-mation flow between you and focus on the correct diagnosis. You might say, "I understand that the exact diagnosis can be very difficult to determine, especially during the first visit. What can we do to help clarify the situation? What might be the most efficient next steps? What is our timing on these next steps?"

Medicine: Art and Science

The art of medicine is to use the doctor's tools (history, physical examination, testing) to assist you and your doctor in the collective determination of the most likely diagnosis and the most appropriate treatment. Many different diagnoses are possible, but likely only one of them is correct. We would all like to think that medicine is a perfect scientific process with predictable outcomes given specific data inputs.

Non-medically trained people may think that the potential list of diagnoses is limited to just a few obvious choices, but in reality, the list can be very long. The list can be so long that the average human brain cannot remember all the possible diagnoses, much less place them into a nice, neat list in descending relevancy of health risk.

This is a biological issue: human cognition is limited by memory constraints. In the case of doctors, they are limited by clinical knowledge and the depth of clinical experience with previous patients. Doctors are humans who cannot possibly know it all and are, in fact, limited by memory and experience. How can we help the physician to improve medical decision making, given these inherent constraints that all humans possess?

The first approach is to ensure that the list of diagnoses within the differential diagnosis is reasonably complete given a specific problem or symptom. The patient can augment the thinking of the physician by aiding in the formulation of the differential diagnosis. To do this, the patient, if possible, and his or her family, should first spend some time researching the condition on the Internet.

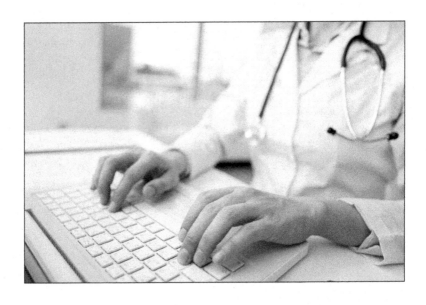

Strategies to Help the Doctor Create a More Complete Differential Diagnosis

Using a search engine, type some of the symptoms into the search box. Look at the diagnoses that are mentioned and read up on each condition. Often within the body of the text on a page for a specific medical condition, there will be a reference to the other diagnoses that should be entertained. Thus begins your own personal list of the differential diagnosis.

The website emedicine.com has a section within each subject chapter devoted to differential diagnosis. You may utilize this as a guide, but it is advised to compile this list on your own. Write down the bullet points: the core aspects of each disease, its symptoms, physical findings, and treatment. Know enough about each condition to be able to speak intelligently with your physician. You should include rare conditions, even though they are unlikely.

The adage "do not believe everything you read on the Internet" is true. However, your goal as a patient is to stimulate thinking and begin the process of building a differential diagnosis. Your use of the Internet is not done with the presumption that all you have learned is correct for your situation; it is simply a stimulator of information and debate to find the truth.

Your physician is your partner in this exercise; you will work together, comparing and contrasting your findings to create the list of differential diagnoses. It is through the vast aggregation of information and clear, detailed communication that you will arrive at an accurate, specific diagnosis. It is important to note that your research may enable you to highlight key factors of the condition, factors you may have missed in your medical history review and that the doctor may have missed in his or her physical exam. Your efforts are an essential ingredient to restore you to full health.

As you are compiling your thoughts using the Internet, keep in mind that your physician may feel defensive when you bring up other potential diagnoses. Draft a short, efficient list with just a few relevant facts that seem to stand out for you. Given that a busy office practice may see a patient every ten minutes, you must be very efficient in your thinking and in your discussion of the differential diagnosis.

Be sure you allow your physician to offer the initial differential diagnosis. Your goal is to add to the strength and accuracy of these initial thoughts, not usurp the process. While showing your list of differential diagnoses, quickly explain that you conducted your own research and reference your sources. When presenting the information, be brief yet cordial. Never forget the reigning principle that you and the physician are a team in a fast-paced ten-minute battle against medical uncertainty. The trophy is uncovering the truth in conjunction with your doctor.

Remain sensitive to the doctor's thoughts and acknowledge their concerns; a successful medical team of patient and physician is a delicate partnership that requires second-by-second nurturing. The steadfast expression of care and diligence by both sides will result in the most likely achievement of successful treatment and health.

Gray Is Okay, Temporarily

As we have discussed, medical conditions are not black and white; they are not clear cut and often not obvious during the first office visit. Even the differential diagnosis may be difficult to formulate during the first visit. In this case, the correct diagnosis will be elusive as well. You must approach the first visit with confidence in the physician as your teammate yet acknowledge that the correct diagnosis may prove a difficult challenge for some time. Given that more work is required, you must expect that monitoring your condition over time will be necessary.

After discussing the potential causes of your illness, it is time to discuss with your doctor how to distinguish between these diagnoses. Evaluating you, the patient, on several serial visits provides invaluable clues since the symptoms and physical findings often change over time. In addition, laboratory tests, EKGs, imaging studies, and specialized examinations may help provide the answer over time as well. Thus labs may be repeated or additional labs may be ordered.

When discussing which tests are to be done, it will be important to think about costs. Should you do comprehensive testing on the first visit or should you undergo the workup in a piecemeal fashion? This will depend on the severity of the situation.

Tests that can determine the likelihood of life-threatening illness should be done first and be done immediately. This may necessitate going to the emergency department of your nearest hospital by car, or in the case of immediately life-threatening illness, by ambulance. However, if the physician determines that your condition is not life threatening, it may be best to conduct only preliminary testing at your first visit. During your follow-up visit, changes in your condition may provide the doctor with clues as to which subsequent tests are needed.

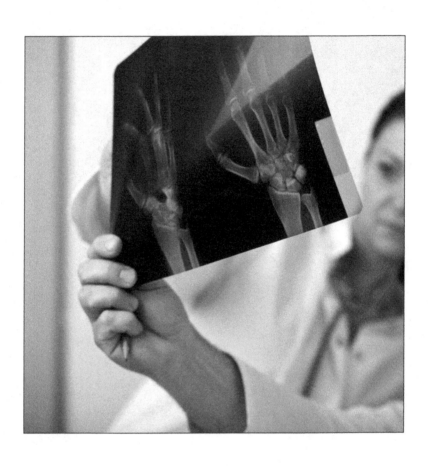

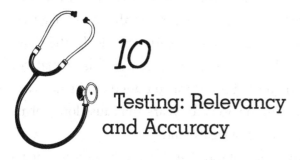

10

Testing: Relevancy and Accuracy

The most important contribution of laboratory testing to your health is: how will the test result change the management of the patient's condition? If the test will not affect the diagnosis or therapy in any way, then it is unnecessary. If you, the patient, have reason to believe that testing may not be needed, you should just ask the simple question, "How will this test affect the diagnosis or treatment?" If the answer does not seem significant, then ask if the physician might be willing to forego ordering the test.

Performing tests has consequences: costs, invasiveness with infection potential, and the perceived need to act on positive tests. Regarding the need to act on positive tests, we need look no further than the debate surrounding the PSA (prostate-specific antigen) test for prostate cancer. Many believe that a high PSA result forces urologists to perform unnecessary biopsies of the prostate with resultant unnecessary surgery.

When your physician suggests a test to help refine the differential diagnosis, it is important to know how accurate that test may be. Let's discuss the example of Lyme disease testing.

Lyme disease testing is known to be inaccurate when it shows a negative result. If the patient actually does have the disease, this is known as a false negative result. In the case of Lyme disease, the very real and common false negative test result is particularly important to understand since the disease can remain in the body for years and cause long-term problems in the absence of treatment.

Given that you understand that the test may show a negative result even if you do carry the disease, it may be appropriate to ask the physician for empiric treatment of Lyme disease. Empiric treatment means that the treatment is provided even though the diagnosis is not proven, per se, by the test or by history and physical examination. This situation requires careful thinking and an open-mindedness on the part of the physician. Today's accepted approach for most all diseases is that physicians must have evidence to support the diagnosis and justify the therapy (known as evidence-based medicine).

Because physicians are taught to prescribe antibiotics carefully and sparingly, it may be difficult for them to make the mental leap to empirically treat Lyme disease, especially when presented with a negative test result. Doctors will only treat empirically if medical history and physical exam provide them with enough evidence to begin treatment.

One form of the Lyme disease rash has a distinctive pattern: a red bull's eye, target appearance. Many physicians will treat empirically given this finding.

Another example of testing inaccuracies is the rapid four-minute in-office test for strep throat. If this test shows a positive result, it is highly accurate; the patient usually does indeed have strep throat. If this test shows a negative result, it is inaccurate in about 10 percent of patients who truly have the disease—a 10 percent false negative result. While waiting for the definitive throat culture to be completed over three days in an outside lab, physicians may prescribe antibiotics empirically in those patients who have a high likelihood of strep throat based on history and physical examination.

Although patients are not physicians, it is in your best interest to know the accuracy of the test you are undergoing so you will be able to judge the accuracy of the diagnosis.

In a directed yet polite way, you must keep pushing for the most accurate diagnosis. The simple questions to ask in order to determine the accuracy of a test are the following: 1) What percentage of the time does a positive test reflect a real condition? (This is a true positive outcome, also known as sensitivity of the test.) 2) What percentage of the time does the absence of a condition result in a negative test? (This is a true negative outcome, also known as specificity.)

If the accuracy of the test is in question, then you must remain especially vigilant in your pursuit of an accurate diagnosis. No diagnosis or therapy is complete until the patient is well with no symptoms.

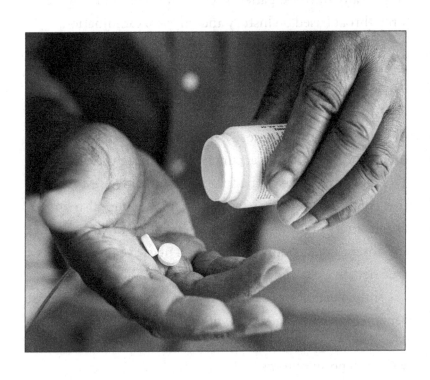

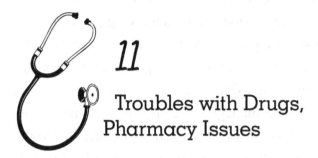

11
Troubles with Drugs, Pharmacy Issues

At the end of your first visit, you will most likely receive a prescription for a pharmaceutical drug to treat your condition. This section provides guidance for you, the recipient of drug therapy.

Prior to the use of computerized medical records, your doctor had to remember drug interactions and remain vigilant to drug allergies. However, the numbers of drug interactions and allergic reactions is so large that no human being can remember them all.

The computer now reminds us of these problems on a case-by-case basis and has lessened the potential for problems with drugs. However, as in all computer use, the system is only accurate if it is fed the correct data. Remember that there are two groups who must have an accurate list of your medications: your doctor and your pharmacy.

Your review of your medications with the medical assistant at the start of your visit hopefully ensures that your doctor sees an accurate list of medications. In regard to your pharmacy, you must remain equally diligent. You must ensure that both your electronic medical record and pharmacy contain the correct medications and allergies logged into their computers. If you are going to be using a new pharmacy, be sure to bring all your medications to the pharmacy as concrete evidence of your present situation.

Pharmacy benefit managers (PBMs) are companies that manage which drugs will be financially supported by your health insurance. Each health insurance company has teamed up with a specific PBM. A PBM becomes involved in your care because they set guidelines as to which drugs they cover for reimbursed costs.

A specific condition might be treated by a very expensive new drug or by an older generic drug. Which drug is the PBM more likely to support? You guessed it: the older generic drug. This is because the PBM will push the physician to write the prescription for the cheaper alternative, which often is the generic version. Many doctors dislike the system because the PBMs are limiting their ability to choose the medicine they think is best for the patient.

You must be aware of PBMs and their effect on doctors and the system of prescribing drugs. Doctors will have strong opinions as to the drug they want to prescribe. Your role in this process is to discuss with the physician the necessity of receiving a new costly drug as opposed to an older cheaper generic drug. You should have this discussion before leaving the physician's office. It is not uncommon for the doctor to prefer the more costly drug; you should be prepared for this scenario.

If you get to the pharmacy and the first choice drug is rejected by the PBM, you have the option of paying out-of-pocket for the drug, or asking the physician to substitute a cheaper, older drug alternative. Time now becomes a factor because the pharmacist can only fill the prescription if it is written in prescription form or verbally agreed to by the physician. Thus, the pharmacist will often call the physician for decisions of this nature. There can be delays associated with this communication, which can adversely affect your health. Your best bet is to discuss the drug choice with the physician prior to leaving the office.

One caveat of this approach is that the doctor will only know which medication is financially most favorable to the patient after the pharmacist has logged the prescription into his computer. Your doctor will not know the PBM-preferred drug at the time he or she writes the prescription.

Therapeutic Interventions Are Not Always Needed

While we are discussing drugs, let us remind ourselves that drugs are not needed for all medical conditions. For example, antibiotics are not needed for viral illness. Wounds that are clean and in good anatomical alignment will heal if simply kept clean and away from contaminants. Indeed, many conditions will be healed by your body itself, without external help. Consistent healthy diet and exercise provide the best backdrop for self-healing. Therapies other than traditional drugs may be effective.

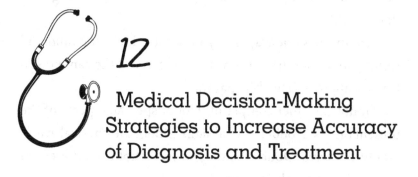

12

Medical Decision-Making Strategies to Increase Accuracy of Diagnosis and Treatment

Let us turn to a review of several thinking processes involved in medical decision making. The central theme of accurate medical decision making is to separate accurate and relevant information from inaccurate and irrelevant information. One of these techniques to obtain medical truths I term "healthy paranoia."

Healthy Paranoia

As the physician works with you on the history and physical exam, they will be constantly looking for significant facts and findings. Each fact and finding will be subject to review by your doctor. Without overtly voicing their reservations, the doctor will be skeptical of each aspect of your interaction. As they are talking to you and examining you, they will be thinking, *what aspects are valid and which are not valid?* This is the essence of healthy paranoia thinking. It takes the form of careful doubting of each data point that arises during your doctor visit.

Just in the same way that your doctor looks for valid and significant data during the visit, you can use the same questioning approach: healthy paranoia.

Doubt the chief complaint. Doubt specific aspects of the present illness. Doubt the vital signs. Doubt the physical exam. Doubt the tests. Doubt the diagnosis. Doubt the differential diagnosis. Doubt the therapy.

Why is this necessary? As has been discussed previously, the nature of medical practice is that many conditions do not lend themselves to an obvious definitive diagnosis or treatment, especially on the first office visit. Thus, it is vital that you, the patient, remain cautious of the physician's diagnosis and remain cautious at all stages of your interaction with your doctor. We advocate that you approach your own situation with a substantial dose of healthy paranoia, just in the same way that your doctor approaches you. Both you and your doctor should employ healthy paranoia thinking as you move through your doctor visit to sharpen critical thinking.

One approach to stimulate healthy paranoia thinking is to say to your doctor, "Our visit together has uncovered a multitude of clinical data. Which of this information appears to be valid and significant to you?"

Let us discuss the simple example of fever as viewed from a healthy paranoia perspective. The patient will often say they have a fever as a component of their illness. Was the fever measured with a thermometer? How accurate is that specific thermometer? Was the fever over 100.4 Fahrenheit (a true fever) or was it the subjective feeling of warmth? The patient says their usual temperature is 98 degrees Fahrenheit, but today the thermometer reads 99 degrees Fahrenheit. Is this minor elevation of temperature significant to uncover the true diagnosis even though this does not fit the definition of a true fever?

In the practical world of your actual office visit, you must not overtly question every data point. This will surely alienate your doctor and result in frustration for both of you. You must support your doctor in their thinking, helping them to examine and identify significant data, using healthy paranoia as a tool.

Remain vigilant in the support of your doctor and their thinking; your approach should never feel oppositional in the eyes of your doctor. Keep your questions to a small number that can be addressed in just a few minutes.

Healthy paranoia is a technique that should not only be used within office visits but also between subsequent office visits. The reason is that you, the patient, will change over time. These changes are often highly significant. Changes might come in the form of worsening symptoms, positive response to therapy, or new testing data that is supportive of a different approach. The accurate diagnosis will only be made by doubting all aspects of the situation and remaining vigilant as to changes that become overtly manifest. This is healthy paranoia in action over time.

Let us examine an example that illustrates the importance of healthy paranoia.

At sixty years old, I experienced the gradual onset of double vision, headaches, and loss of hearing. As a physician who is fully aware of the severity of these symptoms, I was concerned that they could represent a brain tumor etiology. My hope for the definitive diagnosis was a brain tumor called acoustic neuroma since the cure is highly effective surgical removal.

I quickly booked a 9:00 a.m. MRI scan with a neurosurgical appointment at 11:00 a.m. the same day. Following the MRI, I headed over to the neurosurgeon's office. After completing medical history and a physical exam, the neurosurgeon informed me that I did indeed have an abnormal MRI. There was a large mass (an enlarged something) at the base of my brain; this was not a common location for acoustic neuroma. She said quite clearly and simply, "I do not know what this is. I am arranging for you to see a neurosurgeon, ear-nose-and-throat doctor, and an audiologist at a New York City University Hospital this afternoon." Several hours later, after evaluations with twelve different professionals (resident doctors, fellowship-level doctors, and attending doctors), we debated together as we formulated the differential diagnosis.

Some doctors thought that the mass was a vascular tumor (glomus tumor), requiring a trip to the operating room with angiogram and surgical removal. Most doctors could not put the pieces together into a coherent, definitive diagnostic story. Everyone saw the mass as abnormal. Everyone was concerned.

I relay this story to show the high level of complexity and fluidity that can occur in medicine. Extensive discussion within the group and debate of the specifics (healthy paranoia in action) led to the additional conclusion that none of the doctors could specify the correct diagnosis.

This doubting and uncertainty led to the conclusion that

we needed to study the brain with an angiogram performed by CT scan. The CT angiogram would hopefully determine if this mass was a vascular tumor or something else. This noninvasive approach might provide clarity on the medical condition prior to undertaking an operating room procedure with inherent risks (consider noninvasive tests before invasive tests or procedures if possible).

A few days later, the CT angiogram showed an abnormally enlarged vein at the base of my brain, not a tumor. Therefore, no catheter was placed in my brain. The OR was avoided. Unnecessary operative risks were avoided due to careful thinking, healthy debate, and healthy paranoia. Healthy paranoia triumphed. Although the definitive diagnosis was still not clear, we had eliminated the need for the knife. (We will discuss the outcome of this case further on in this book in the chapter "Difficult Diagnosis.")

Doubt everything, and the truth comes out. This is the working thesis of healthy paranoia. Perform your own internal debate as it relates to your specific condition. Ask questions of your physician to ensure he or she has considered all possible scenarios. Remain diligent to support your doctor at all times in the discussion.

Within your questions, be careful with your words. Trust and partnership with your physician must reign supreme. It is best to ask your questions once the physician has provided a definitive diagnosis or discussed the differential diagnosis. Utilizing your own differential diagnosis list, you might ask politely, "Have you considered X disease as a possibility?" It may additionally be a good idea to comment that you understand how difficult diagnostic and therapeutic decisions can be, as you are aware of how many variables can affect the outcome. With this demonstration of respect in place, your doctor will be more open to your inquiries. This will allow you to continue to build a strong partnership rooted in trust.

If you simply doubt, doubt, doubt, you are using negative terms and emanating only negative energy to your physician. Negative feelings cannot be allowed into the patient-doctor partnership; they are counterproductive. Always remain upbeat and supportive of your doctor, even while discussing your doubts. This is an art you must master prior to challenging your doctor with doubting questions.

The art of the medical visit is to be able to convey your sense of trust in the physician yet aim for truth, even when it is elusive. Every test, every reevaluation, every change in medical condition is a positive step in the right direction, even when it may appear to be a step in the wrong direction. Ensuring that patient and physician take the time that is necessary to arrive at the correct diagnosis is of critical importance in medicine. Healthy paranoia within the setting of a positive patient attitude will result in medical truth and the best possible medical outcome.

Stressed: In or Out?

All of us have stress in the course of our daily lives. This is the normal state of living life. The central question is the following: is stress the exact cause of my medical condition? We all know that stress accompanies our medical conditions. Is it playing a parallel part or is it playing the central role?

In certain straightforward situations, stress is clearly the culprit. For example, consider a fast heart rate only felt while flying in an airplane. When flying, the patient's heart beats at greater than one hundred beats per minute. When on the ground, the heart beats between sixty and one hundred beats per minute. Clearly the stress and fear of flying are causing the rapid heart rate.

If you feel stressful in certain specific situations and you have bodily symptoms at these times (such as stomach pain, acid reflux, sweating, headaches), then perhaps stress is the root cause. Unfortunately, the symptoms often do not start and stop in exact relationship to the presence or absence of a stressful situation. For example, a new college student may have persistent headaches that they never had before starting college. However, since they are most always at college, the headaches persist throughout the fall semester and even when home on break. We cannot say for sure whether or not the only cause of these headaches is stress.

Many patients come to their doctor in a very stressful state. The doctor's job is to be highly observant so they notice the stress. After evaluating the patient, perhaps the doctor thinks through the differential diagnosis and places stress at the top of the list. Since stress is highly prevalent and often causes disease states, it is tempting to see stress as the cause, the etiology (doctor term for cause). The problem with this approach is that other organic causes of the symptoms may be overlooked. The treatment may therefore not be effective, and the patient may experience prolonged suffering.

Let us take hyperthyroidism as an example. Hyperthyroidism causes fast heart rate, panicky feelings, feelings of warm skin flushing, weight loss, and stressful feelings or thoughts. If a patient demonstrates these symptoms and hyperthyroidism is detected by a simple blood test, proper treatment will likely resolve all of these symptoms. If stress, per se, is thought to be the root cause, the symptoms will continue. Hyperthyroidism has been overlooked because it was not considered during the evaluation as part of the differential diagnosis.

In order to combat the temptation to label stress as the root cause of our symptoms, we must ask hard questions of our doctor.

"Is it possible that my symptoms could be caused by something other than stress? What is the differential diagnosis of my situation? Could we place stress at the bottom of the list and consider all other causes first?"

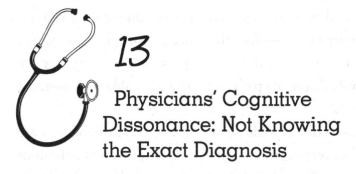

13

Physicians' Cognitive Dissonance: Not Knowing the Exact Diagnosis

Not knowing the exact accurate diagnosis is not a comfortable situation for physicians. Yet this is a daily, commonplace event. Given the multiplicity of diagnostic possibilities and the inability to figure out the puzzle within the first visit, the physician is left with substantial cognitive dissonance: the uncomfortable feeling that the all-important medical truth is elusive. The inability to identify the correct diagnosis can lead to adverse outcomes for patients. Deteriorating conditions can lead to death in the absence of the correct diagnosis and therapy. The pressure is very real to find the truth, yet delays will occur due to the time required to do the workup through testing and reevaluation of the patient over time.

One can readily understand the paramount need for an emergency department at a hospital that can access testing, imaging, and specialists with a fast turnaround time.

Most patients are treated at a doctor's office where testing turnaround times are measured in days versus hours at a hospital. Indeed, most of the time, this is appropriate: most patients' conditions are non-emergent and do not require a trip to the hospital. Therefore the office physician is confronted with a situation in which the diagnosis and therapy may not be identified, yet the patient is uncomfortable with ongoing symptoms.

Understandably, high levels of cognitive dissonance are felt in the everyday interactions with patients on a continuous basis in the office setting. The doctors would like to do all tests on a stat (immediate) basis, but this is not possible outside the hospital. The high cost of performing tests at hospital emergency departments prohibits the routine use of the facility for non-life-threatening conditions.

To feel better about the cognitive dissonance, the doctor may unconsciously use two techniques. These two common techniques are the "first-thoughts effect" and "explaining away symptoms." I write about these techniques, as they became evident in my own medical evaluations throughout the course of several years.

First-Thoughts Effect

The first-thoughts effect is the notion that the first diagnosis coming into the mind of the physician is likely the most accurate diagnosis because it is a common entity and easily fits the symptoms. The ability to latch onto the first diagnosis as the true diagnosis is a good feeling for the physician because it fits the symptoms and is a reasonable first guess. In addition, the thinking process consumes less time and cognitive energy.

It is much more difficult to think of all the possibilities first (develop the differential diagnosis), then work back to the true diagnosis by eliminating each one individually. In this case, the physician must force him or herself to hold back the obvious diagnosis and think through the subtleties of the less obvious diagnoses. This approach is not easily done by human beings in any profession.

Patients can encourage physicians to combat the first-thoughts effect by posing a very simple question in a kind and receptive manner: "We understand that the diagnosis at the top of your list is the most likely because it is common, but are there any other diagnoses that we should be thinking about at this time? We are open to your thoughts."

Explaining Away Symptoms

The second technique to calm cognitive dissonance is "explaining away symptoms." In this approach, the doctor rationalizes a cause for each symptom that does not fit his initial working diagnosis.

For example, a patient comes to the doctor for symptoms of a rapidly beating heart along with severe anxiety. The doctor latches on to the diagnosis of anxiety as the working diagnosis since the patient has had anxiety symptoms for many years. The patient is an adolescent and has never had any cardiac issues.

Fully knowing that these symptoms could be the result of anxiety or an intrinsic electrical defect of the heart, the doctor may rationalize that the cause is not intrinsic heart because the patient has a long history of anxiety, is young, and has no known risk factors for cardiac disease.

As in all human beings, it feels better to the doctor when the patient could be thought of as having a panic attack, a common condition that is not life threatening. Given that anxiety and mental health issues are major determinants of daily life for most humans, panic attack is a very real possibility for the true diagnosis. Panic attack is a convenient diagnosis, because it does not need critical intervention; the physician feels good about this situation.

However, a physician who believes panic attack to be the true diagnosis has not considered that an intrinsic heart condition called supraventricular tachycardia (known as SVT) also causes a very rapid heartbeat. This SVT is a pure heart problem with abnormal electrical excitation within the heart; it is not related to the brain or the neurological system.

Medical problems are not simple: cause and effect of a disease may be hard to differentiate. For example, anxious feelings similar to an anxiety attack accompany a heart beating out of control due to SVT. Thus, a patient with a rapid heartbeat could be experiencing either pure anxiety or could have anxiety as a result of an electrical problem of the heart.

The natural tendency for most human beings is to look first for the most common and simple explanation for a symptom like anxiety (first-thoughts effect described above). As a way to justify our quick thinking, we as doctors explain away the symptoms, thinking that pure cardiac disease is not common in adolescents with no known heart disease.

The treatments for these two causes of anxiety are vastly

different. Should the correct diagnosis not be uncovered, the patient might suffer needlessly for a prolonged period of time.

So how does a patient guard against these situations, the first-thoughts effect and explaining away symptoms? Our approach relates to the section above concerning the differential diagnosis. You and the physician together can formulate a differential diagnosis list. For the patient, the key item is to ask, "What are the different possibilities for the diagnosis and how do we separate out the differences between them?" This simple question ensures the construction of a complete differential diagnosis list that results in a clear action plan. In doctor jargon, we call this the workup.

The workup sets the foundation for eliminating improbable diagnoses and identifying the diagnosis that is most accurate. As aforementioned, the workup can take the form of 1) additional detailed physical exam, 2) laboratory tests (blood, urine, other bodily fluids), 3) imaging (x-rays, CT scans, MRI scans) and, 4) examining the patient over time as regards to response or lack of response to therapy.

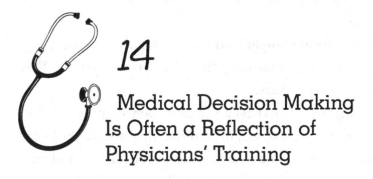

14

Medical Decision Making Is Often a Reflection of Physicians' Training

It should be no surprise to any patient that a surgeon loves to cut and sew. It should be equally no surprise that an internist loves to ponder medical facts. Each caregiver has an approach to their work that utilizes a set of skills and strengths they have learned in residency training. Thus, when you are burdened by a condition and faced with choosing a specific caregiver, it is imperative that you understand the caregiver's strengths in order to maximize your chances of arriving at an accurate diagnosis. As you undergo the office visit and workups, you should continue to consider their background and the inherent biases that influence their thought processes.

Many caregivers are proud of their training and personal approach to diagnosis and therapy. If you ask, they will likely enjoy explaining the benefits of their approach.

Let's look at a few specialties in detail in regards to their type of training and potential for bias. These are overly simplified generalizations; however, they may give some starting thoughts and questions as to the orientation of a specific caregiver.

Internists are taught to think in a highly analytical way. They are experts at building the differential diagnosis. They are analytical thinkers.

Family physicians have all of the responsibilities and challenges of an internist, yet, in addition, they are taught to pay attention to the whole patient: body, mind, family, and relationships. They care for patients of all ages and all conditions.

Pediatricians are similar to internists and family physicians, except their focus is on infants through adolescence. Childhood diseases and therapies are often quite different than adult medicine.

Psychiatrists are taught to look at the emotional side of life with special attention to the efficacy and side effect profile of pharmaceuticals that treat these conditions. They enjoy untangling the thoughts of the mind.

OB-GYN physicians are multifaceted in their approach. They have a love of both medical and surgical treatments of the female reproductive system and enjoy delivering babies.

Ophthalmologists primarily address conditions of the eye and eyelids. Thus their diagnostic and therapeutic worldview is encompassed within a very small area. Their surgeries take place in this same small area and are often performed using a microscope. They are highly detail oriented.

Orthopedists are carpenters whose medium is not wood but bone. They enjoy working with bone: sawing it, placing screws into it, reinforcing it with metal braces. Orthopedists enjoy noninvasive treatments as well and will exhaust them prior to suggesting surgery.

In addition to knowing a doctor's specific type of residency training, it is important to know if they have any specific biases or approaches.

As an example of a unique approach, let us discuss the case of my family's local dermatologist. This physician is an Ivy League-trained allopathic physician who has done extra training in nutritional supplement therapies for dermatological conditions. One of my children had an acne condition that was addressed by all modern medicine therapies, including potent antibiotics, without resolution of the condition. This dermatologist used her knowledge of an alternative nutritional approach called muscle response testing, in which she prescribed natural, whole-food nutritional supplements. My child's acne condition resolved in a matter of weeks.

Choosing a physician is an important step in the pursuit of optimal health. We propose the following approach: 1) keep an open mind as to all potential caregivers; 2) identify primary care doctors or specialists that are best suited to address your condition; 3) research on the Internet the nearby physicians in these fields: read their webpage, review their educational background, their experience, and their strengths; 4) consider inherent biases and skills based on their background that could influence medical decision making and therapy. Be especially vigilant to novel approaches to diagnosis and therapy. Discuss with current patients their experience with the physician.

15
Post-Visit Conclusions and Next Steps

Now, let us imagine you have just left the physician's office. How comfortable are you as to the accuracy of the diagnosis and the appropriateness of the treatment? Do you have a sense of the differential diagnosis and the relative level of potential danger within each one of these diagnoses? Where are you in the process of arriving at the definitive diagnosis and receiving accurate treatment? End (definitive diagnosis has been given, along with treatment)? Middle (definitive diagnosis not clear despite complete workup and differential diagnosis)? Beginning (differential diagnosis in early development)?

What does your doctor think are the next steps to resolving the diagnosis problem? Second round of detailed workup? Referral to specialist?

If your diagnosis and treatment appear to be accurate and effective, then both you and the doctor will be happy with the outcome.

If, however, the diagnosis is not clear, nor is the therapy

effective, it may be appropriate to entertain thoughts of novel and robust approaches to the problem.

The next section will aid you in developing a strategy to approach these difficult diagnoses.

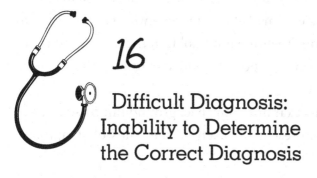

16

Difficult Diagnosis: Inability to Determine the Correct Diagnosis

You have been to your primary care doctor several times for the same problem without resolution. They have referred you to specialists in your town. Those specialists have referred you to university hospital physicians. Even the university physicians cannot understand why you have this problematic condition.

You continue to have symptoms that compromise your daily life. The answer is elusive; the cause of the condition remains unknown. Frustration starts to consume your usual positive daily energy. Months go by without any progress; your frustration levels are building.

The absolute necessity of determining the correct diagnosis is essential because understanding the underlying mechanism is the key to understanding the correct therapy. If the diagnosis is incorrect, the therapy will be incorrect. These words appear to be obvious caveats, but the detailed processes to delineate the medical truth are the essence of improving one's medical condition.

Although the numbers of patients whose true diagnosis remains elusive is small, it is a supremely important situation for that person. Their life is on hold. In the next sections, we will provide several specific details as to how to overcome these obstacles.

First let us examine some background information as to how diseases present themselves: the "silos of symptoms" situation.

Difficult Diagnosis: Silos of Symptoms

Let us examine the situation where a patient has symptoms relating to multiple different body parts during the same illness. For example, a patient might have joint aches, headache, fatigue, fever, loss of left-sided facial muscle function, and rash. If the primary care physician is unable to determine the correct diagnosis, the patient might visit a rheumatologist to address the joint aches, a neurologist to address the headaches/facial muscle dysfunction, and a dermatologist to address the rash.

The seemingly unrelated nature of multiple symptoms relating to multiple organ systems is what we call "silos of symptoms." The symptoms seem unrelated since they occur in different organ systems. However, the cognitive leap required to reach this patient's correct diagnosis is to realize that all these symptoms are indeed the result of Lyme disease. This one disease is causing multiple symptoms to surface as a result of impaired functioning of multiple organ systems.

Each specialty physician has been trained to evaluate a specific body part of the patient. As a young doctor in specialty training, we may indeed learn how the specialty organ system interacts with the rest of the body. However, the day-to-day practice exposes specialists to common single-organ-system diseases. Rarely does the specialist have to address a complex constellation of symptoms relating to different bodily organs for a single patient.

The silos of symptoms situation is a major obstacle to uncovering the correct diagnosis. Each specialist directs their attention to the areas of medicine they know well. Unless they consult reference books and look for ways to connect the silos, they may miss the bigger picture. You, the patient, can ignite this necessary secondary level of thinking by asking the simple question: "Is it possible that all these different symptoms are related in some way to a single diagnosis?" This is a question you will want to ask your primary care physician during your first visit for a specific illness.

Let us examine a particularly difficult pediatric example of silos of symptoms.

A friend of mine has a child who exhibits multiple symptoms relating to multiple organ deficiencies: heart, kidney, and skin. Our local pediatricians were unable to identify the underlying condition, and the patient was referred to a children's hospital in Boston. The child then underwent evaluation by multiple specialists over the course of an entire day at the Boston facility. At the end of the day, the specialists met together in one room and were able to pinpoint a very rare condition. Despite the existence of the silos of symptoms challenge, the doctors were able to identify the correct diagnosis. The key to unlocking the correct diagnosis was to have all specialty physicians discuss the case in one location at one time.

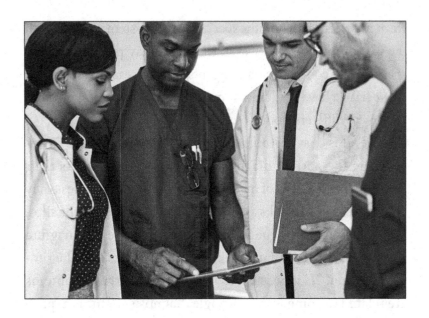

Specialists who work in a community setting will often send the primary care physician a detailed report of their history, physical exam, workup, and diagnosis. It is rare for specialists and primary care doctors to sit together in one room at one meeting to discuss one patient. As in the pediatric case discussed above, the face-to-face presentation of the case and detailed discussion is commonly done only at university teaching hospitals. We will discuss advantages of teaching hospitals in the section below entitled "Difficult Diagnosis: Local University Hospitals."

One more essential point regarding silos of symptoms: your primary care doctor is in a unique position to connect the silos with the resultant correct diagnosis.

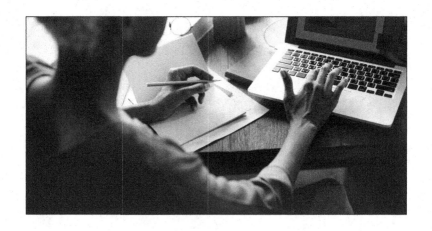

Difficult Diagnosis: Internet Techniques for Online Textbooks and Online Medical Research Papers

The first tactic to be used in a difficult diagnosis situation is for you, the patient, to perform Internet searches within online medical textbooks to develop a more complete differential diagnosis list.

The first set of searches should be done using online medical textbooks, such as www.emedicine.com because the textbook authors have performed a thorough overview of each specific diagnosis. The chapter for each diagnosis includes sections on presenting symptoms, physical findings, workup, therapy, and differential diagnosis. The easiest way to start the search is to use your symptoms as the search terms.

For example, a patient with numbness of the arm could conduct a search using the term "paresthesias" (the medical term for this condition). The reason that we start with symptom names as our search terms is that many symptoms are indeed diagnostic terms as well. Once we begin to read about a specific diagnosis that seems to be related to our symptoms, we can then read that chapter's list of differential diagnoses. The chapter devoted to each one of the diagnoses on this much larger list can then be reviewed for appropriateness to the present condition.

In summary, use the following steps for the Internet textbook approach: 1) search online textbooks using your specific symptoms as the search terms; 2) review each chapter and write down each of the differential diagnoses listed within each chapter to build a grand list of a differential diagnosis; 3) review each chapter from the differential diagnosis grand list and determine its appropriateness to your condition; 4) print out each diagnosis chapter and bring it to your next office visit.

Internet Search: Original Research Articles and Review Articles

The second tactic for difficult diagnosis Internet search is to examine the online medical research papers written by experts in the subject you are searching. This is much harder than Internet searching of textbooks, as more medical knowledge is required.

In many cases, the research papers are written by MDs and PhDs that have devoted their lives to a specific disease. Their knowledge of the disease is often highly detailed with multiple ongoing research projects. Consequently, their research publications are likely to be very detailed and thorough.

Your best approach to search the medical literature is to use www.pubmed.gov.

There are two types of articles to examine: original research articles and review articles. Original research articles can be identified by their emphasis on a hypothesis and experimental method mentioned in the abstract at the beginning of the paper. Review articles are identified by a notation in the abstract that the article is a review article and by the large number of papers referenced by the author (often hundreds of references to prior papers).

When performing an Internet medical literature review,

first look for review articles that focus on the working diagnosis as a way of gaining a robust overview of the subject. A review article is similar to a textbook chapter in that it discusses all the major concepts related to a specific diagnosis. However, it is more detailed than a textbook chapter because it features summaries of specific experiments of the focus area.

Second, find original research articles regarding the working diagnosis. Begin to develop a list of authors who have written several articles within a specific diagnosis. In most areas of medicine, there will be a few clinicians that have developed a supremely advanced level of knowledge in that area. Your goal is to locate these individuals for your specific diagnosis.

The clinicians who write original articles must review the relevant literature in detail in order to compose the article. Thus, in addition to knowing the background information regarding the diagnosis, they are also thinking of new concepts for their research efforts. Their daily work is to examine cutting-edge concepts of your disease area.

Difficult Diagnosis: University Hospital Specialist

The most common progression of doctors' visits for a difficult diagnosis patient is the following: 1) primary care provider, 2) local specialist, 3) university hospital specialist. Let us examine the advantages and disadvantages of the university hospital specialist.

Why is the university specialist so adept at difficult diagnosis? The daily activities of the typical university physician offer a unique educational environment in medicine: 1) many of their patients come from far distances and have a difficult diagnosis themselves (thus these clinicians are challenged by the most difficult cases on a regular basis); 2) daily or weekly interactions with young doctors-in-training both at the bedside (clinical rounds) or in conference (grand rounds); and 3) participation in clinical or basic science research that requires fundamental knowledge and creative thinking in these areas. A university-based physician is most often a specialist whose emphasis is to evaluate the most unique and difficult cases.

Despite the advantages of a university specialist, most medical conditions can be appropriately addressed much closer to home in highly appropriate and effective avenues at the primary care physician office. Primary care is also likely to be much cheaper than a university private practice. Additionally, university practice may not be covered under insurance plans. If the insurance company will not cover the cost of the university visit, you will be responsible for the entire cost of the care. Thus, be sure to take advantage of all local resources prior to university care. Should you need university care, first place a call to your insurance company to determine which benefits are applicable to your situation.

If your medical need is still unmet after visiting your primary care doctors and local specialists, a trip to the regional university practice is warranted. How can you determine which physician will be the best one for you to see?

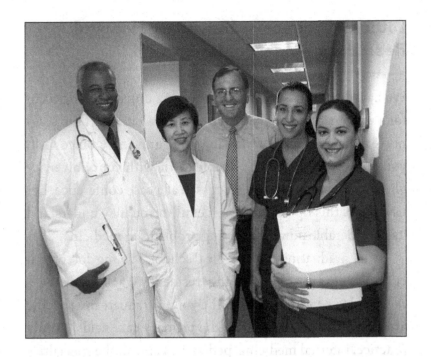

First locate the university/medical school's website online and examine the physician profiles for the specific department you are interested in. Then call the practice's reception desk, explain the situation, and ask which physician has the most experience in the area most similar to your situation. Having done your research, you can ask about any names the receptionist does not mention. By doing your homework prior to the telephone call, you are most likely to identify the most qualified and appropriate physician. If the front desk personnel seem unsure of who would be most appropriate, ask to speak with the nurse in charge. They will be very knowledgeable as to physician experience, knowledge, and specialized expertise.

Difficult Diagnosis: University Hospital Resources: Case Conference

We have just discussed how to choose a university physician for a university private practice office evaluation. If the diagnosis remains unclear following your university office visit, you may discuss another possible tactic with your university physician: your case to be discussed at a case conference. Let us discuss this option in more detail so you may understand its considerable power in solving problems in medicine.

After graduating from medical school, a young doctor will enter the next phase of training: residency. Each residency is designed to educate and train the young graduate in a specific area of medicine: think of all the primary care fields (family practice, internal medicine, pediatrics) and all the specialties of medicine (ophthalmology, neurology, general surgery, orthopedics, etc). Each one of these fields has multiple hospital training sites in the United States; each residency program is composed of one or more hospitals, usually with one anchor university hospital responsible for coordinating all the training.

Each week, a four-hour conference is conducted at the university hospital in which residents are lectured on medical topics in addition to other educational activities. One of these four hours is dedicated to the presentation and discussion of a complex clinical patient: hence the term case conference. The patients presented often portray rare or difficult to diagnose conditions.

Case conference is the ideal place for your difficult

diagnosis case to be presented because many university and local physicians attend these conferences with the common goal of solving the case.

Let us take as an example my own difficult diagnosis case discussed earlier in this book. My symptoms experienced over five months included headaches, right-sided hearing loss, and double vision on left lateral gaze. As you recall, my local neurosurgeon referred me to a New York City university team of specialists. Through noninvasive CT angiography, they determined that the mass in my brain was not a tumor but rather a large vein. However, they could not understand how my symptoms could stem from this large vein. They were perplexed as to the cause of the symptoms, and thus no therapy could be proposed. There was still no closure, no definitive answer, and no definitive therapy.

My response to this situation was to call up the Department of Neurology at a different teaching hospital in Connecticut. I requested an evaluation by the most appropriate neurologist and asked that my case be discussed at the weekly case conference the next week.

A week later, my case was presented at the case conference with more than sixty physicians in attendance: neuroradiologists, neurologists, and neurosurgeons. They uniformly agreed that the large vein at the base of my brain did not explain my symptoms and was unrelated to my condition. Their working hypothesis was viral encephalitis. It was recommended that I undergo testing to confirm this diagnosis: lumbar puncture to test the cerebral spinal fluid for virus.

On the day I was intending to have a lumbar puncture, the

headaches, hearing loss, and double vision began to resolve. Subsequently, all the symptoms resolved.

This case illustrates several points: 1) multiple universities and multiple teams were necessary to uncover the correct diagnosis since no one physician could identify the cause; 2) a less invasive diagnostic approach was able to provide significant data; and 3) knowledge of healthy paranoia techniques and university hospital resources was the key to unlocking the truth.

Another case within my family illustrates the power of multiple physicians debating a medical case in case conference. One of our family members had experienced numbness of his left hand for several months. His local internist and neurologist ran tests for chemical abnormalities, including an MRI of his brain, but no diagnosis could be determined. His case was presented at case conference in front of forty neurologists (both attending neurologists and resident neurologists) at a local university hospital. One of the neurologists asked what the results of the lumbar puncture (fluid that surrounds the brain and spinal cord) had shown. This test had been overlooked in prior workups. When this test was subsequently performed, it showed lymphoma cancer cells within the fluid. Thus the diagnosis of central nervous system lymphoma was made. The correct diagnosis helped this patient to prepare for his short remaining lifetime and enjoy his last few months with our family as best as possible.

Difficult Diagnosis: Identification of National Expert

Following your Internet searches of online textbooks, review articles, and original research, you should have developed an extensive differential diagnosis and have printed out all relevant articles. You have discussed these with your primary care physician, your local specialist, and perhaps your university specialist. If you and your doctors are still unable to pinpoint the correct diagnosis, then it is time to consider evaluation by a national expert clinician.

Accessing a National Clinical Expert

Examine your Internet articles. Divide them into three groups: 1) textbook chapters, 2) review articles, and 3) original research articles. The original research articles are the ones we think you should review in order to locate a national expert.

Look at the names of the authors carefully. If you notice an "MD" after their name, it is likely that they evaluate and treat patients at a university clinical practice. Once you have identified a clinician who writes articles highly relevant to your area of interest, you now need to locate their clinical office to schedule an appointment.

Find their affiliated medical institution on the first page of the original research article. Then, using an online search engine, look up the institution and the relevant department, paying particular attention to the list of faculty/clinicians. Read the biography of the clinician you seek and ensure that he/

she is appropriate for you. On the faculty page, there should be a phone number listed that can be used for setting up appointments. If you are unsure how to get in direct contact with the clinician's office, call the relevant department chairman's office. They will quickly direct you to the appropriate private practice front desk.

The goal of this second Internet-based technique is to put you in front of the most experienced caregivers in a specific area of medicine. However, there are some important considerations: you will likely have to travel a very far distance to reach them. In addition, your insurance company may not be willing to reimburse you for the cost of the office visit. This could result in a very expensive consultation. How can you ensure this visit will be productive and worth the extra expense?

First, we advise that you call the clinician directly to provide them with preliminary information. This conversation will be discussion of the most basic symptoms, prior workup, and the fact that no other clinician has been able to specify the correct diagnosis.

After reaching a receptionist at the private practice office, politely introduce yourself, briefly explain you have a difficult situation that requires further consultation, and request to set up a two-minute phone call with the physician. Once on the line with the clinician, introduce yourself and state that you located them through reading their articles online. Explain that the purpose of this call is to ensure that they are willing to evaluate you and that they are, in fact, a highly experienced clinician in this area.

Next provide a very basic one-minute summary of your situation. This is the presentation of your condition as discussed previously: the 1) chief complaint, 2) history of the present illness, 3) past medical history, 4) the workup, and 5) working diagnosis to date.

After this quick presentation, you might ask: "Would it be appropriate for me to come see you as a patient given your status as an expert in the area?" This permits the clinician to provide their initial thoughts on the following information: 1) relevance of their knowledge, 2) confirmation of relevant tests that have already been done and suggestions for testing to be done with your primary care doctor prior to travel, and 3) names of other clinicians that may be more appropriate and worth contacting.

Most important to the clinician is that you are not asking for them to practice medicine or provide an accurate diagnosis over the phone. You are not even asking for their impressions of the differential diagnosis.

You are simply asking an expert how best to proceed in order to gain the truth behind your medical situation.

If the clinician agrees to evaluate you as a patient, your next call should be to your insurance company. Explain that no physician (primary care, local specialist, university physician) has been able to definitively diagnose you. You are requesting that they cover the cost of the visit even if the expert clinician is not listed within their network. You will gladly provide them with a letter demonstrating the necessity for an expert evaluation.

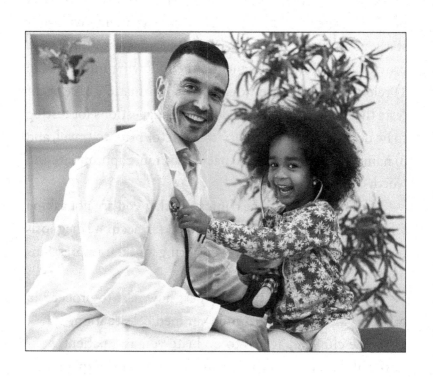

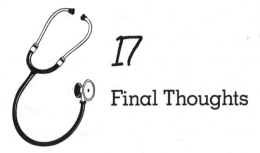

17
Final Thoughts

Medicine is complicated. The process of the medical visit is complicated. Most importantly, medical decision making is complicated.

Attaining best outcomes requires diligent care and nurturing by both the physician as well as you, the patient. Your efforts are critical to help your physician navigate this complex medical situation.

Prepare for the medical visit by writing down your own notes of chief complaint, history of the present illness, past medical history, past surgical history, present medications, allergies, social history, and family history. Practice your presentation of these components by speaking them out loud to yourself prior to the visit. Present them to the medical assistant or nurse and again in great detail to the doctor. Do your homework on the background of the physician prior to arrival. Perform your Internet search (textbook chapters, review articles, original research) of the differential diagnosis. Write down your preliminary list of the differential diagnosis. Print all articles and bring them to the visit.

During the process of the visit, utilize techniques of familiarization with the staff/physician, healthy paranoia, discussion of differential diagnosis, and discussion of therapies. Understand the relevancy and accuracy of testing. Discuss new, expensive therapies versus older generic therapies. Ask effective, coherent, and concise questions. Above all, bond with your physician. See them as your friend, your advocate, your teammate, and your fully invested partner.

See your doctor as you see yourself: a human being who cares deeply for your health but needs support and careful consideration. Help your physician to help you create an exceptional doctor's visit. The goal of accurate diagnosis and effective therapy is a healthy life for you and your loved ones.

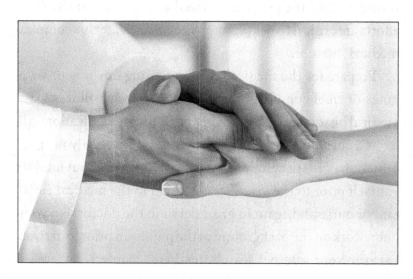

About the Author

Kilbourn Gordon III, MD majored in psychology at Swarthmore College. Not knowing what his future might hold during senior year in college, he took the advice of two friends who advised him to study medicine. Having not studied science during college, he then went on to study premedical requirements at the University of Vermont. After attending New York Medical College, he completed residencies in both emergency medicine and ophthalmology. Along with a great team of physicians, he helped to establish the Emergency Medicine Residency Program at the California College of Medicine, Irvine, CA, where he was assistant professor of Emergency Medicine. For several years, he was the director of the Examination of the Patient Course, the medical students' first exposure to patients by conducting history and physical examinations. He won two awards for outstanding teaching of medical students during this time. He lives with his wife, Caroline Britton Gordon, in Darien, CT and is clinically active in urgent care medicine at the present time.

Communicating with the Author

Comments, critiques and proposed improvements are always welcome. If you experienced a clinical situation with significant positive outcomes that can help other patients please submit a detailed description for possible inclusion in the second edition of Med School 101 for Patients. Please e-mail us at the following address: kgordonmd@medschool101forpatients.com.

Addendum: Case Presentation Template

This template will help you prepare for your visit. Please fill in the blanks and bring a copy of the completed form to your visit. Practice the presentation out loud before leaving for your office visit. Be prepared to present your case initially to the medical assistant who first interviews you and once again when you are with the doctor.

Chief Complaint:

I am a ___ (age in years)-year-old _____(male or female) with a ___ (numbers of hours, days, or months) history of _____(two- or three-word description of the chief complaint).

History of the Present Illness:

The following are descriptions of my condition:

_____

(dull ache, electric pain, radiation of pain, comes and goes, constant, etc).

It is associated with several other symptoms:

_____

(fever, chills, vomiting, diarrhea, abdominal pain, malaise, sore throat, etc).

My condition is made worse by the following:

_____

(exercise, bending, specific movements, etc).

My condition is improved by the following:

_____

(rest, non-weight bearing, acetaminophen, ibuprofen, other medications, etc.).

My prior workup with Dr. _____ showed the following:

_____

(physical findings, laboratory results, imaging results)

Past Medical History:

_____

(diabetes, hypertension, heart attack, stroke, gout, surgeries, etc. with year of onset)

Past Surgical History

_____

(type of surgery and year performed)

Allergies:

_____

(specify medication and symptoms, year of onset)

Medications:

_____

(specify each medication, the milligrams, and the frequency)

Social History:

_____

(smoking history: packs per day for how many years; marital status)

Family History:

_____

(presence of cancer, heart disease, cancer, stroke, diabetes in siblings, parents, or grandparents)

Addendum: Essential Questions

"What are the most likely things that could be causing my illness? Are any of these causes particularly dangerous? Is there a critical time factor for any of these conditions?"

"I understand that the exact diagnosis can be very difficult to determine, especially during the first visit. What can I do to help clarify the situation? What might be the most efficient next steps? What is our timing on these next steps?"

"Our visit together has uncovered a multitude of clinical data. Which of this information appears to be valid and significant to you?"

"Is it possible that my symptoms could be caused by something other than stress? What is the differential diagnosis of my situation? Could we place stress at the bottom of the list and consider all other causes first?"

"We understand that the diagnosis at the top of your list is the most likely because it is common, but are there any other diagnoses that we should be thinking about at this time? We are open to your thoughts."

"What are the different possibilities for the diagnosis and how do we separate out the differences between them?"

"Is it possible that all these different symptoms are related in some way to a single diagnosis?"

"Would it be appropriate for me to come see you as a patient given your status as an expert in the area?"

Bibliography

Websites

www.medscape.com
www.emedicine.com
www.epocrates.com
www.pubmed.gov

Books

Bickley, Lynn S. *Bates' Guide to Physical Examination & History Taking. 12th Edition.* Lippincott, Williams & Wilkins, 2016.

Bickley, Lynn S, *Bates' Pocket Guide to Physical Examination and History Taking, 8th Edition.* Lippincott, Williams & Wilkins, 2016.

Dains, Joyce E. *Advanced Health Assessment & Clinical Diagnosis in Primary Care, 5th Edition.* Mosby, 2015.

Fortin, Auguste H. *Smith's Patient Centered Interviewing: An Evidence-Based Method, 3rd Edition.* McGraw-Hill Education/Medical, 2012.

Henderson, Mark. *The Patient History: Evidence-Based Approach, 2nd Edition.* McGraw-Hill Education/Medical, 2012.

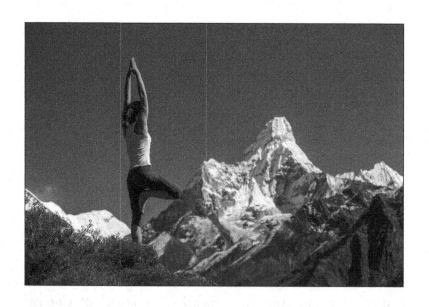

Printed in the United States
By Bookmasters